CU00704080

Anti-Inflammatory Diet Cookbook

Dinner Recipes

42 Healthy and Delicious Recipes to Reduce Inflammation and Boost Autoimmune System

Gena Pemberton

Table of Contents

Introduction

An anti-inflammatory diet should contain a recommended daily intake of 2,000 – 3,000 calories, 67 grams of fat and 2,300 mg of sodium. Fifty percent (50%) of those calories should come from carbohydrates, twenty percent (20%) should

come from protein and the remaining thirty percent (30%) should come from fat.

You can get carbohydrate-rich foods from eating whole-wheat grains, sweet potatoes, squash, bulgur wheat, beans and brown rice.

On the other hand, your intake of fat should come from most types of fish and any foods cooked in extra-virgin olive oil or organic canola oil. You can get protein from soybeans and other whole-soy products.

This diet prohibits fast food or processed food in any part of the meal. This also means a restriction on pork, beef, butter, cream and margarine. The antiinflammatory diet should also contain less processed sugar for diabetics and low cholesterol (though Omega-3, which is found in a variety of fish, is a good cholesterol) for people with heart problems.

Benefits of an anti-inflammatory diet

One of the benefits of an anti-inflammatory diet is that it uses fresh foods with phytonutrients that prevent degenerative ailments from occurring. The diet plan also produces cardiovascular benefits; thanks to the inclusion of the Omega-3

fatty acids. These fatty acids aid in preventing complications in the heart and reducing the levels of "bad" cholesterol and blood pressure.

Another benefit of the anti-inflammatory diet is that it is diabetic friendly. As

this diet restricts processed sugar and sugar-loaded meals and snacks, it works

perfectly for patients who are suffering diabetes. While the diet does not

substantially reduce weight, it decreases a patient's likelihood of suffering from

obesity. This is due to the inclusion of natural fruits and vegetables, and the restriction of meat and other processed foods.

1. **<u>Creamy Rice Pudding with Blueberry Compote</u>**

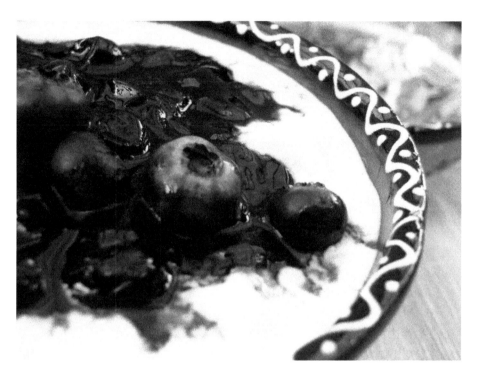

Prep Time: Time: 1 Hour

Serves: 8 – 10

Ingredients:

- Rice Pudding:
- 1 ½ cup Basmati Rice – brown, organic
- 2 ½ cups Water
- 1 pinch Salt
- 4 cups Rice Milk
- ½ cup Demerara sugar
- 2 tbsp. Potato Starch

- Cinnamon powder – to taste
- For the Blueberry Compote:
- 3 cups fresh, organic Blueberries
- ½ cup Sugar
- ¼ cup Water

Directions:

1. Add the rice and water to a medium saucepan and bring to a boil.
2. Add the salt and gently stir the contents. Once boiled, reduce the heat to low, and simmer the rice.
3. Fold the rice in gently until all the water is fully absorbed.
4. Add to this, the brown sugar and 2 pinches of cinnamon powder and mix. Add the rice milk and continue to cook for about 10 minutes.
5. Dissolve the potato starch in a few tablespoon of water and add to the rice mix.
6. Allow the mixture to simmer on low heat until it thickens and remove from the heat.
7. Allow to cool, and transfer to a bowl. Place the bowl in the fridge and allow it to cool.
8. In a small saucepan on medium heat, crush the blueberries to a small pot and add the sugar and water.
9. Bring to boil and allow it to simmer. Remove from the heat after a minute or two.
10. Once chilled, serve with the warm Blueberry compote.

2. Savory Sweet Carrot Muffins

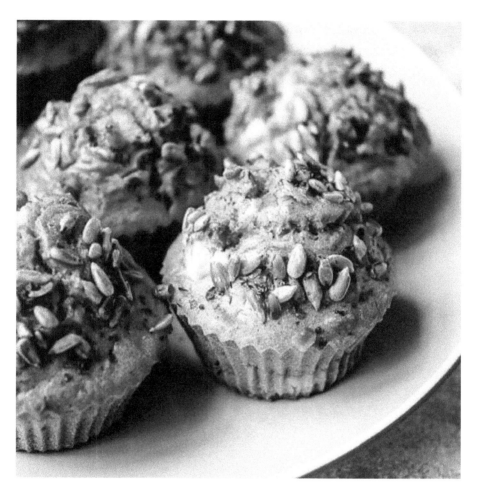

Prep Time: 30 Minutes

Serves: 10 – 12

Ingredients:

- 1 ½ cup Milk / Rice Milk
- 2 small Eggs
- 4-5 tbsp. Canola Oil

- 3 cups Quinoa/Gluten-free flour
- 4 tbsp. Demerara Sugar
- 2 tbsp. Flaxseed meal
- 2 tsp Baking Powder – gluten free
- 1 pinch Salt
- 1 pinch Cinnamon powder
- 3 medium Organic Carrots – grated
- ½ cup Raisins

Directions:

1. Preheat oven to about 400°F. In a bowl, whisk the egg with the oil and milk.
2. In another bowl, mix the dry ingredients, and add it to the wet mix, stirring gently till well blended.
3. Add the grated carrots and the raisins to the batter and fold the mixture.
4. In a muffin pan, grease the muffin moulds or line with muffin cups. Fill the cups till about 2/3 full.
5. Bake this in the oven for about 20 minutes. Remove from the oven and place on a wire rack to cool. Enjoy!

3. Fresh Millet Pancakes with Fruit Compote

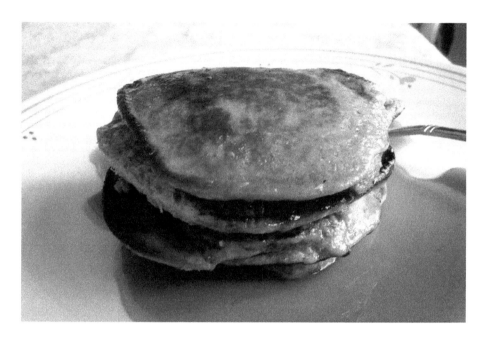

Prep Time: 45 Minutes

Serves: 3 – 4

Ingredients:

- 1 ½ cup Millet grains
- 3 tbsp. ground Millet flour
- 2 cups Skimmed milk
- 1 pinch Salt
- 100 ml of Carbonated Water
- 2 tbsp. Sugar
- ½ cup Yogurt – non-fat, plain
- 2 Eggs, lightly beaten
- 500 gm dried, pitted organic Plums

- 3 cups Water
- 3 tbsp. Apple juice

Directions:

1. In a medium saucepan, add the milk, millets and salt and bring to a boil over a medium heat.
2. Once it comes up to a boil, bring the heat down to a simmer and cover for 20 minutes until the milk is absorbed by the millets.
3. Gently mash the millets to a paste, and fold in the yogurt, eggs and sugar with the millet flour. Add the carbonated water to make the batter to your desired consistency.
4. In a separate bowl, add the cherries to warm water and allow it to soften.
5. Preheat a non-stick skillet on a medium heat, and spray with vegetable cooking spray. Ladle the batter onto the skillet using a spoon and shape into a pancake disk.
6. Gently cook each side for about 3-4 minutes until golden brown and flip over to repeat the same for the other side.
7. In another saucepan, add the plums, sugar and water and bring to a boil.
8. Add the apple juice and allow to simmer for about 15 minutes until the plums are soft.
9. Plate the pancakes and serve with the compote.

4. **Probiotic Cantaloupe Smoothie**

Prep Time:: 15 Minutes

Serves: 1 – 2

- Ingredients:
- 1 medium sized Cantaloupe – deseeded and coarsely chopped.
- 1 medium pack Probiotic Yogurt
- 1 Vanilla bean – deseed
- 2 tbsp. Organic Honey
- Crushed Ice

Directions:

1. Add all the ingredients to a blender and blitz until smooth.
2. Pour into a tall smoothie glass and garnish with a mint leaf and slice of lime.
3. Serve chilled.

5. <u>Crepe de Quinoa et Applesauce</u>

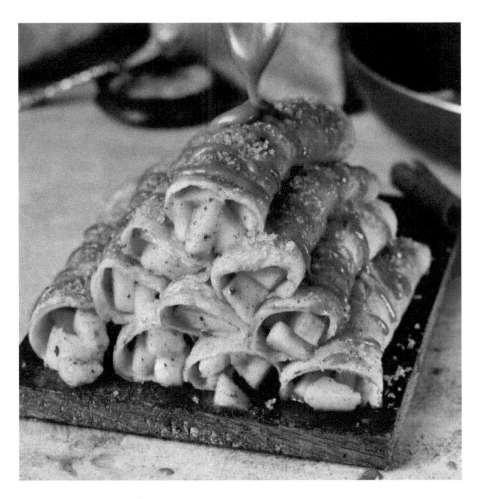

Prep Time:: 30 Minutes

Serves: 10 – 12

Ingredients:

- 1 ½ cup Organic Quinoa flour
- ½ cup Organic Tapioca flour
- 1 pinch Baking Soda powder

- 400 ml Sparkling water
- 4 tbsp. Canola oil
- 1 small tsp Cinnamon powder
- 4 cups Organic Applesauce – unsweetened

Directions:

1. Mix both the flour in a medium bowl with the baking soda. Add the cinnamon powder and mix gently.
2. Stir in the canola oil and carbonated sparkling water to this, until the batter reaches the desired consistency.
3. Check for lumps, and stir till smooth.
4. Place a non-stick skillet on medium heat, add a few drops of oil and spread it to grease the skillet.
5. Pour about 3 tablespoon of the batter and rotate the skillet to
6. spread it to form the crepe.
7. Cook until the side is a light golden brown and flip over gently.
8. Keep making crepes until the batter runs out.
9. Serve the crepes hot with the applesauce.

6. **Raspberry Apple Crumble**

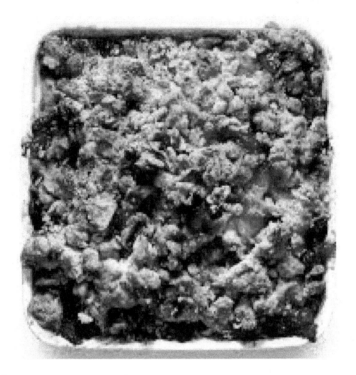

Prep Time:: 1 Hour 15 minutes

Serves: 4-6

Ingredients:

- 6 large cooking Apples – thinly sliced
- 1 cup Raspberries
- 2.5 cups Apple Juice
- 2.5 cups Rolled Oats
- ¼ cup Butter (or) Margarine
- 3 tbsp. Brown Sugar (Demerara)
- 1.5 tsp Cinnamon powder
- 1.5 tbsp. Clove powder

Directions:

1. Preheat the oven to 350°F. In a greased baking dish, arrange the sliced apple and raspberries and pour the apple juice to cover this.
2. In a bowl, mix the rolled oats, sugar and spices to form a rough flour. To this, add the butter and mix in with your fingers to make the crumble topping.
3. Layer the crumble topping onto the laid out apples and raspberries until they are covered with a uniform layer.
4. Bake for about 45 – 60 minutes.
5. This crumble can be served hot or cold.

7. **Butter Almond Cookies**

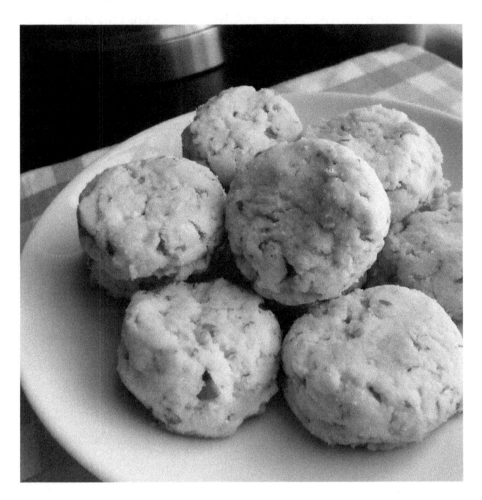

Prep Time:: 30 Minutes

SERVES: 6 – 10

Ingredients:

- ½ cup Organic Coconut oil / Organic Butter
- ¾ cup Organic Coconut Sugar
- 1 Egg

- 1 teaspoon Vanilla Extract (or) 1 whole Vanilla Bean (slit and extract the seeds)
- 1.5 cups Almond Flour
- 1 cup Almond Butter (Crunchy or Smooth)
- 1 pinch Sea Salt
- ½ cup Coconut Flour

Directions:

1. Preheat the oven to 350°F.
2. In a bowl, add the coconut oil, almond butter and sugar and mix well using a spatula.
3. Add the egg, salt and vanilla and mix together until smooth.
4. To this, add the almond flour and the coconut flour and mix well to form a firm dough.
5. Allow to set for 10 minutes, then use a tablespoon to scoop out a small ball and place onto a greased cookie tray.
6. You can use a fork to flatten the dough – this also gives the dough a nice design if you press down in a criss-cross pattern.
7. Place as many cookie balls as you can and flatten then so that they don't touch each other.
8. The dough does not expand, so there's no worry about loading the tray to full.
9. Place the cookie tray in the oven, and bake for 10-12 minutes at 350°F. Remove the tray from the oven and allow the cookies to cool.

8. Pocket-sized Buttermints

Prep Time:: 2 hours 10 minutes

SERVES: 6 – 10

Ingredients:

- ½ cup Butter (Pasteurized) (or) ½ cup Organic Cold Pressed (Virgin) Coconut oil
- 4 Tbsp. Organic Raw Honey
- 10 - 14 drops Peppermint essential oil (or)
- 5 – 10 drops Peppermint oil
- Yield: Approximately 60 small sized Buttermints.

Directions:

1. Keep the butter at room temperature. In a bowl, add all the ingredients and stir to combine. Add peppermint oil or extract to suit taste.
2. Add the mixture to a pastry bag, and squeeze out button sized servings onto a parchment lined baking tray, and place in the fridge for about 2 hours till the mints set.
3. You can then transfer this to a storage container that can be kept in the fridge.
4. For the recipe with coconut oil, mix all the ingredients and pour the batter onto a parchment lined baking tray.
5. As this batter will be softer than the butter batter, you won't be able to pipe this into button sized servings.
6. Place this in the fridge for 2 hours; allow setting, and simply cutting into squares.
7. Transfer this to the storage container and keep in the fridge.

9. **Strawberry Gelato**

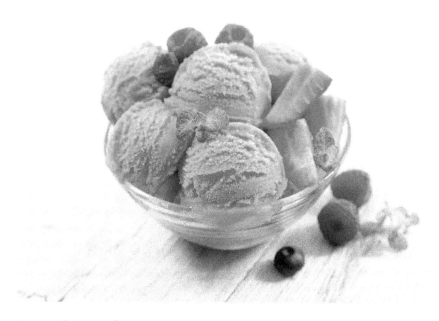

Prep Time:: 5 hours 30 minutes

Serves: 6+

Ingredients:

- ¼ cup Butter/Coconut oil (or) 1 cup Heavy Cream
- 4 Egg yolks
- 2 cups Milk / Coconut milk (if lactose intolerant)
- ½ cup Maple Syrup/Honey/Stevia Tincture
- 2 cups Fresh Strawberries, stemmed with tops removed and pureed
- A pinch of sea salt
- Lemon Zest – optional (Half tsp).

Directions:

1. In a saucepan, add the milk and cream and bring to boil. After this, allow the mix to simmer, while constantly stirring for about 4-5 minutes.
2. In a blender, whisk the egg yolk, honey and salt till you get a smooth and creamy mix.
3. Continue to whisk on a low speed, slowly adding the warm milk mix.
4. You have to be very careful at this stage or you can end up with cooked eggs.
5. Once the milk has been added, carefully empty the contents into the saucepan over a medium low heat, and stir constantly till the mix starts to thicken.
6. To this, add the pureed strawberries and lemon zest and combine thoroughly.
7. Allow the mixture to chill in a refrigerator for a minimum of 4-5 hours till it is completely cooled down. Leaving it overnight in the fridge will make a deeper, intensive flavor.
8. Once the mixture is completely chilled, add this to an ice-cream maker to make the gelato.
9. In case you don't have an ice-cream maker, you can make this in the blender/food processor by simply freezing the mixture for 2-3 hours, blitz it in the blender till smooth and then refreezing for another 2-3 hours.

10. <u>Fudgy Sweet Potato Brownies</u>

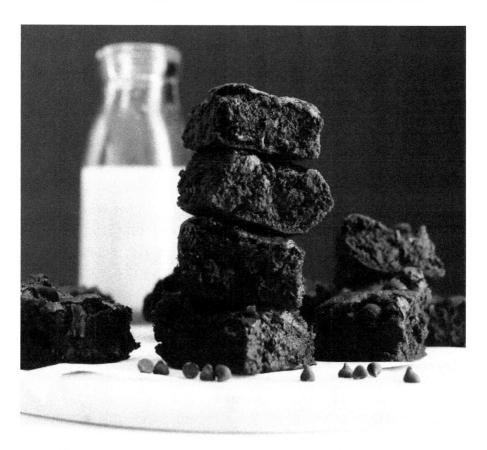

Prep Time:: 40 Minutes

Serves: 4

Ingredients:

- ¼ cup cold pressed Coconut Oil
- ¾ cup unsweetened Cocoa Powder
- ½ cup Pastry Flour (Whole Wheat preferred)

- 1 pinch Baking Powder
- 1 pinch fine Sea Salt
- 1 cup Coconut Sugar
- 1 cup Sweet Potato Puree
- 1 Tbsp. ground flaxseed meal + 3 Tbsp. cool water
- 1½ tsp pure vanilla extract

Directions:

1. In a small bowl, add the flour, salt and baking powder and mix well.
2. Place a saucepan on a low flame and melt the coconut oil. Stir in the cocoa powder until the entire mix is smooth.
3. Add the sweet potato, flax seed meal, water, sugar and vanilla to a large bowl and whisk thoroughly. You might need to keep at it for a bit as the coconut sugar can take a bit of time to dissolve.
4. Add the cocoa and coconut oil mixture to the large bowl and keep whisking.
5. Add flour to this and keep whisking till smooth and the batter has a glossy appearance.
6. Lightly grease an 8"x8" glass baking pan with coconut oil, and preheat the oven to 350°F.
7. Pour the batter into the pan, and bake for 20 to 30 minutes.
8. The top should appear hard and baked. When you stick a butter knife into the center, it should come out smooth with a few moist crumbs.
9. Note: The total baking time will depend on what type of sweet potatoes you use.
10. In case you use canned puree, it can take a bit longer as they have higher moisture content.
11. Stir in the flour till smooth, scrap into the prepared pan.

11. <u>**Millet Pancakes with Prune Compote**</u>

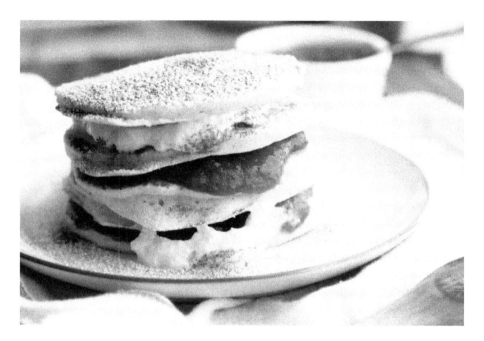

Yields 4: servings

Ingredients

- 2 tablespoons apple juice
- 2 tablespoons brown sugar
- 2 cups water
- 16 oz. organic dried plums pitted and softened.
- Vegetables cooking spray
- 2 tablespoons millet
- 1 egg, lightly beaten
- 1/3 cup plain non-fat yogurt
- 1 tablespoon sugar
- ½ cup carbonated water
- 1 teaspoon salt
- 2 cups skim milk

- 1 cup millet

Directions:

1. Place millet, milk, and salt in a medium saucepan and bring to boil, then simmer covered for 20 minutes.

2. Stir in the sugar, carbonated water, egg, yogurt, and millet flour.

3. Over medium heat, preheat a large non-stick skillet and spray with vegetable cooking spray.

4. Ladle batter into the skillet and spread with a spoon to form 3-inch pancakes. Fry until golden brown. Flip over and continue cooking for 4 minutes.

5. Place prunes, sugar, and water and apple juice in a saucepan and bring to a boil.

Reduce the heat and simmer for 12 minutes or until the prunes are tender.

6. Let the prune completely cool for a few minutes then serve on pancakes

12. <u>Anti-oxidant Muffins</u>

Yields: 6 servings

Ingredients

- 1 large egg
- ¼ cup almond milk
- 1 cup blueberries
- ¼ teaspoon salt
- 1/3 cup pecans, chopped
- ½ teaspoon baking powder
- 1/3 cup brown sugar
- 1 cup whole-wheat flour

Directions:

1. Preheat your oven to 350 degrees Celsius.

2. Combine sugar, flour, pecans, powder, and salt. In a separate bowl, lightly beat the egg and almond milk. Then proceed to combine the dry and wet ingredients.

3. Pour the batter into your paper muffin cups then proceed to bake for 40 minutes and transfer the muffins to a cooling rack.

4. Serve warm.

13. <u>Nettle Crepes with Raspberries</u>

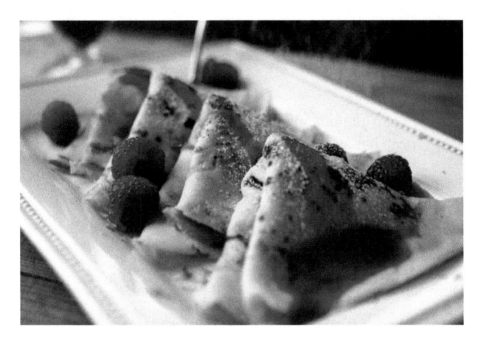

Yields: 2 servings

Ingredients

- Fresh raspberries
- Vegetable cooking spray
- 1 teaspoon salt
- ¼-teaspoon white pepper
- 7 oz. young nettle shots, blanched and chopped
- 1-cup all-purpose flour
- 2 cups organic milk
- 2 organic eggs

Directions:

1. In a medium bowl, beat the eggs; add nettle, milk, pepper, and salt. Whisk until well combined.

2. Preheat a large nonstick skillet over medium heat, and then spray with vegetable cooking spray.

3. Pour out 3 tablespoons of batter onto the skillet, rotating the skillet very quickly until

the bottom evenly coats. Cook the crepe for 2 minutes or until light brown. Flip and

cook for another 30 seconds then remove from the skillet.

4. Repeat step 3 until all the batter is finished.

5. Serve crepe with mashed raspberries.

Sauces, Condiments And Dressings

14. **Anti-Inflammatory Turmeric Dressing**

Yields: 1 serving

Ingredients

- ¼ cup extra virgin olive oil
- 3 tablespoons of vinegar
- 2 teaspoons of honey
- 1 teaspoon of dried dill weed
- ¼ teaspoon garlic powder
- ¼ teaspoon ground black pepper
- ½ teaspoon fine sea salt
- 1 teaspoon of ground turmeric

Directions:

1. Place all the ingredients in a shaker bottle with a tight fitting lid and shake well.

2. Pour and toss over your favorite salad greens.

15. <u>Anti-Inflammatory Salad Dressing</u>

Yields: 4 servings

Ingredients

- 1/8 teaspoon black pepper
- 1/8 teaspoon salt
- 1/8 teaspoon mustard powder
- ½ teaspoon curry powder
- ½ teaspoon fresh minced ginger
- ½ teaspoon ground turmeric
- 1 tablespoon raw honey
- 1 tablespoon ACV
- 2/3 cup unsweetened cashew milk, dairy free
- 1 tablespoon chia seeds
- ¼ cup raw cashews

Directions:

1. Place the chia seeds and cashews in a spice grinder and grind into powder.

2. Place the cashew-chia mixture in your blender with about ½ of the cashew milk. Blend until smooth.

3. Add the remaining cashew milk, honey, vinegar, agave, turmeric, ginger, salt, mustard, and pepper. Puree for 60 seconds

4. Chill for 30 minutes for maximum thickening and melding of the flavor. After the 30 minutes, briefly blend before pouring atop your salad.

16. <u>Creamy Turmeric Sauce</u>

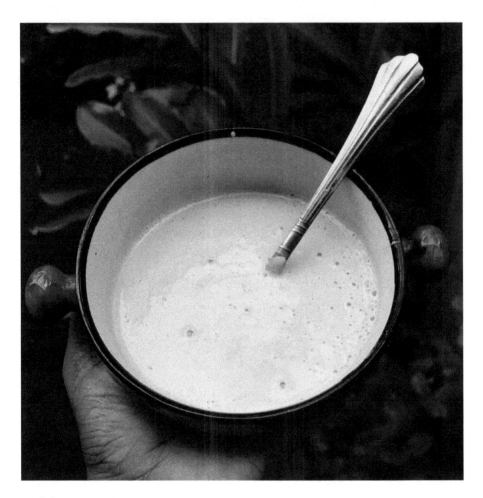

Yields: 2 servings

Ingredients

- 1 teaspoon onion powder
- 1 teaspoon garlic powder
- 1 teaspoon turmeric
- 2 teaspoons salt

3 cans 13.5 oz. coconut milk

Directions:

1. Pour coconut milk into a saucepan.

2. Add all the spices, mix well and bring to boil.

3. Let it simmer for 30 minutes to thicken the sauce. The longer it simmers, the thicker it will become and the stronger the sauce.

17. __Cherry Coconut Porridge__

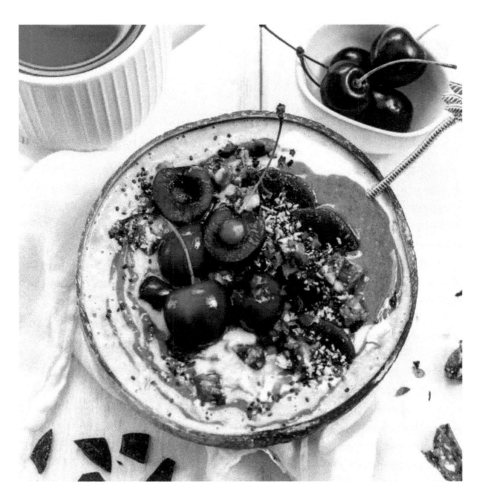

Ingredients

- 1.5cups oats
- 4 tablespoons chia seed
- 3-4cups of coconut drinking milk
- 3 tablespoons raw cacao
- pinch of stevia
- coconut shavings

- cherries (fresh or frozen)
- dark chocolate shavings
- maple syrup

Directions:

1. Combine oats, chia, coconut milk, cacao and stevia in a saucepan.

Bring to a boil over medium heat and then simmer over lower heat until oats are cooked.

2. Pour into a bowl and top with coconut shavings, cherries, dark chocolate shavings and maple syrup to taste.

18. <u>Feel-Good Pineapple Smoothie</u>

Ingredients:

- 1 ½ cups frozen pineapple chunks
- 1 orange, peeled
- 1 cup coconut water
- 1 tablespoon finely chopped fresh ginger (or 1/4 teaspoon ground ginger)
- 1 teaspoon chia seeds, plus extra for garnishing
- 1 teaspoon McCormick Ground Turmeric
- 1/4 teaspoon ground black pepper

Directions:

1. Add all ingredients to a blender. Pulse until smooth.

2. Serve immediately, garnished with extra chia seeds if desired.

19. <u>Greek Yogurt Cheesecake Cups</u>

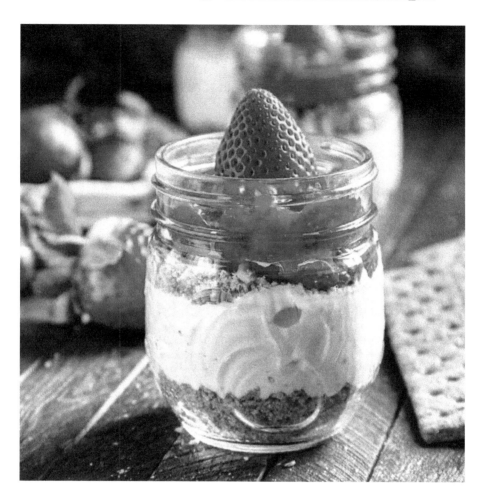

Ingredients

- 2 cups semisweet chocolate chips
- 2/3 cup reduced-fat cream cheese
- 1/4 cup powdered sugar
- 1/3 cup plain Greek yoghurt
- 1/2 tsp fresh orange zest

Directions:

1. Pour one and a half cups of the chocolate chips into a glass bowl

and melt in the microwave for 2 minutes, stopping to stir every 30 seconds, until the chocolate is smooth and completely melted.

2. Stir in the last half-cup of the chocolate chips and mix together until all the chocolate is smooth and glossy.

3. Drop a spoonful of the melted chocolate into 8 cupcake liners. Use a spoon to spread the chocolate into an even layer and bring the chocolate up the sides of the liners to help keep the filling in the cup.

4. Put the chocolate cups in the fridge while you mix the filling. In a medium bowl, beat the cream cheese with a 1/4 cup of the powdered sugar. Taste. If you want it a little sweeter, add some more powdered sugar and mix until there are no more lumps.

5. Mix the greek yoghurt and orange zest into the cream cheese

mixture.

6. Once the chocolate cups have set, take them out of the fridge and drop a spoonful of the cream cheese filling into each one. Spread the filling into an even layer. Place the cups back in the fridge for about 5 minutes to let the cheesecake filling firm up a little bit.

7. Take the cups back out, stir the rest of your melted chocolate (reheat for a few seconds if you need to), and drizzle the melted chocolate over the top of the cheesecake filling. Gently spread the chocolate over the filling, then put the cups back in the fridge for 5-10 minutes until the chocolate has hardened. Remove from liners and serve.

20. **Greek Yogurt Berry Parfait**

Ingredients

- 1 cup nonfat plain Greek yoghurt
- 1/2 cup sliced strawberries
- 1/2 banana
- 2 tbsp nonfat granola
- Natural sweetener, such as stevia

Directions:

1. Mix natural sweetener with non-fat plain Greek yoghurt until desired sweetness is reached.

2. In a glass, alternately layer strawberries, Greek yoghurt and bananas.

3. Sprinkle granola on top, chill and serve.

21. <u>Fluffy Vegan Blueberry Quinoa Pancakes</u>

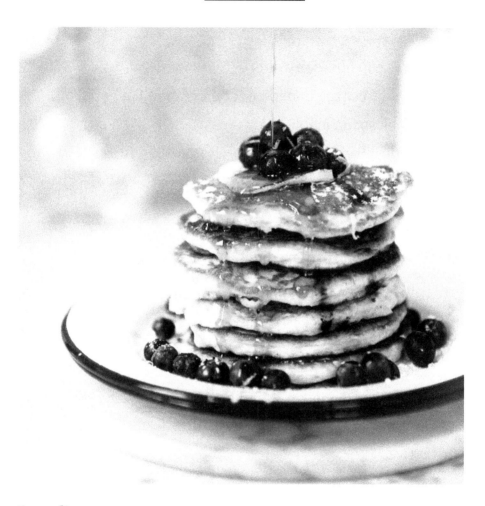

Ingredients

- 2 flax eggs (2 tablespoons flaxseed meal + 6 tablespoons water)
- 1 cup q uinoa flour (I like to toast mine)
- 1/2 cup almond flour

- 2 tablespoons arrowroot starch
- 2 teaspoons coconut flour
- 2 teaspoons baking powder
- 1/2 teaspoon sea salt
- 1 1/4 cup non-dairy milk
- 3 tablespoons almond oil (or other light flavoured oil)
- 1 tablespoon maple syrup
- 1 cup blueberries (fresh or frozen, but frozen will turn them bluer!)

Directions:

1. Preheat a griddle over medium heat.

2. Whisk together the flax and water and set aside to gel.

3. In a large mixing bowl, whisk together the flours, baking powder and salt.

4. Beat together the flax eggs, milk, oil and syrup then pour into the dry and mix until smooth batter forms. Fold in the blueberries.

5. Lightly grease your griddle with nonstick cooking spray or coconut oil. Ladle ¼ cup of batter onto the griddle and repeat until you have filled your pan. Cook the pancakes until small bubbles begin to form around the edges, about 2 – 3 minutes.

6. Flip and cook for another 1 – 2 minutes longer until the other sides are golden brown. Repeat until no batter remains.

7. Serve warm with fresh berries (or fruit of choice) and pure maple syrup.

22. Maple, Walnut and Flaxseed Pancakes Recipe

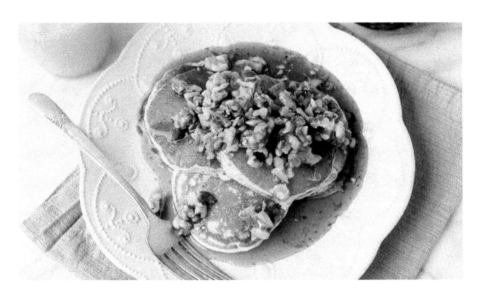

Ingredients:

- 1 cup all-purpose flour
- 1/4 cup flaxseed meal*
- 1/4 cup finely chopped walnuts
- 1 1/2 teaspoons baking powder
- 1/2 teaspoon baking soda
- 1/2 teaspoon salt
- 1 1/4 cups reduced-fat (2%) buttermilk
- 1/4 cup pure maple syrup
- 1 large egg
- 1 tablespoon (or more) vegetable oil
- Additional pure maple syrup

Directions:

1. Whisk flour, flaxseed meal, walnuts, baking powder, baking soda and salt in medium bowl. In a separate medium bowl, whisk buttermilk, 1/4 cup maple syrup and egg. Add buttermilk mixture to dry ingredients and whisk until incorporated.

2. Brush a large nonstick skillet lightly with vegetable oil and heat over medium heat. Working in batches, add batter to skillet by scant 1/4-cupfuls.

3. Cook, until bubbles appear on surface of pancakes and undersides, are golden brown, about 2 minutes.

4. Turn pancakes over and cook until golden on bottom, about 2 minutes. Brush skillet lightly with vegetable oil as needed between batches. Transfer pancakes to plates. Serve with additional maple syrup.

23. **Avocado Chocolate Mousse**

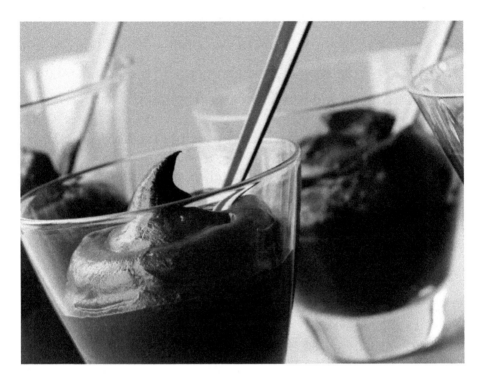

Ingredients

- 3 ripe avocados
- 6 oz plain Greek yoghurt
- 1 bar dark chocolate
- 1/8 cup unsweetened almond milk
- 1/4 cup finely ground espresso beans
- 2 tbsp raw honey
- 1 tsp vanilla extract
- 1/2 tsp sea salt
- 1/4 cup sugar

- 1/4 cup cocoa powder

Directions:

1. Mix all ingredients together, then puree in blender.

2. Set in fridge to cool.

24. <u>Chocolate Cake with Vanilla Frosting</u>

Ingredients:

For Cake:

- ½ teaspoon baking soda
- 12 free-range eggs
- 1 cup virgin coconut oil
- ½ cup raw cacao powder
- 1 cup coconut flour
- 1 cup pure maple syrup
- 4 tablespoons vanilla extract
- 1 teaspoon salt
- For Vanilla Icing:
- 2 cans of full-fat coconut cream (liquid drained from can)
- 4 tablespoons pure maple syrup
- ½ teaspoon almond extract
- 4 teaspoons vanilla extract

Directions::

For Cake:

1.Add all of the ingredients to a blender and blend on high for 30-45 seconds,

allowing the eggs to froth.

2.Pour batter evenly into two 6 inch cake pans.

3.Bake at 350 degrees for 30 minutes or until cake passes the toothpick test.

4.Cool before frosting.

For Vanilla Icing:

1.Chill coconut milk in the fridge for at least 6 hours, preferably overnight.

(Recipe will not work without it being chilled.)

2.Without shaking the cans, remove them from the refrigerator.

3.Carefully open the cans of coconut milk and scoop the thickened cream into

a bowl.

4.Add the pure maple syrup, vanilla extract, and almond extract to the heavy

coconut cream.

5.Mix thoroughly with a hand mixer... will take 3-5 minutes.

6.Place in refrigerator and allow icing to cool to thicken until it meets the tex-

ture you most prefer. Frost the cake.

25. **<u>Blueberry Peach Cobbler</u>**

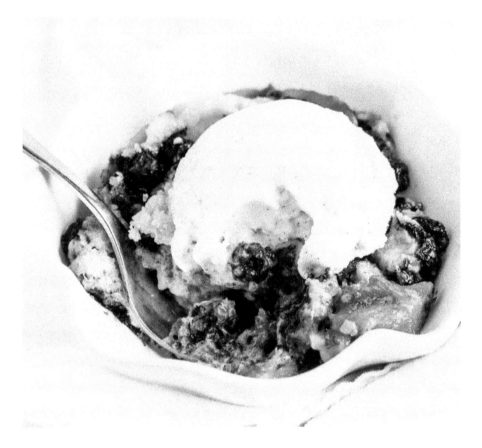

Ingredients:

Filling:

- 2 pounds organic or freshly thawed from frozen peaches, roughly chopped
- 2 cups organic fresh or frozen blueberries
- ¼ cup pure maple syrup
- ½ teaspoon ground cinnamon

- 1 teaspoon vanilla extract

Crumb Topping:

- 1 ½ cups walnut halves
- 2 tablespoons pure maple syrup
- ¼ teaspoon sea salt
- ½ cup shredded unsweetened coconut
- 1 tablespoon melted coconut oil

Directions:

1.Preheat oven to 350 degrees.

2.In a large saucepan, over medium heat, combine the peaches, blueberries, maple syrup, vanilla, and ground cinnamon. Stir until the syrup comes to a boil, then allow mixture to simmer until the syrup has thickened a bit and the peaches are fork tender. Turn off the heat and allow the pot to sit while you make the crumble.

3.To make the crumble, place the walnuts and shredded coconut in the bowl of a large food processor. Process until a crumbly texture is formed, then add the maple syrup, coconut oil, sea salt, and almond extract. Process again, until a sticky and crumbly mixture is formed.

4.Pour the peach filling into a 9-inch square or round baking dish, then sprinkle the crumble over the top evenly.

5.Bake at 350 degrees for 15 minutes, or until the top is lightly golden. Serve warm.

26. <u>Watermelon Popsicles</u>

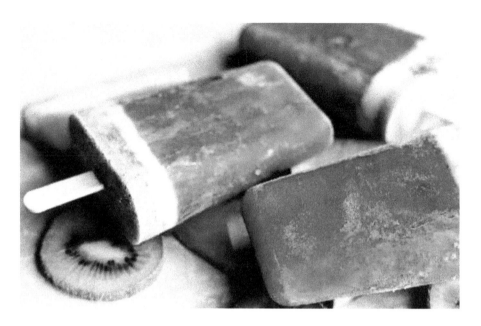

Ingredients:

- 1 ½ cups sliced watermelon
- 4 reusable Popsicle containers

Directions:

1.Blend the slices of watermelon in a blender (you may need to add a tiny amount of water to get the watermelon blended).

2.Pour watermelon juice into reusable Popsicle containers.

3.Freeze overnight.

27. **<u>Peppermint Patties</u>**

Ingredients:

Chocolate:

- 8 tablespoons coconut oil, melted
- 4 tablespoons raw cacao powder or cocoa powder
- 4 tablespoons maple syrup

A few grains of salt

Peppermint Patty:

- 2 cups unsweetened shredded coconut
- ½ teaspoon (food-grade) peppermint essential oil or
- 1 teaspoon of peppermint extract
- 4 tablespoons maple syrup
- 6 tablespoons hot water

Directions:

1.Line a 12-count muffin tin with paper or silicone muffin liners.

2.In a food processor, blend all ingredients together for the chocolate. (It will be on the liquid side of textures.)

3.Pour chocolate into the base of each muffin tin, just covering the bottom, and leaving about ⅓ of the chocolate in the mixing bowl.

4.Allow chocolate in the muffin tin to cool in the freezer.

5.In a food processor, add the coconut, peppermint, maple syrup, and hot water. Blend until everything is well combined.

6.Remove chocolate from the freezer.

7.Add a tablespoon (or so) of coconut mixture on top of the chocolate, pressing gently.

8.Drizzle remaining chocolate over the tops of the coconut.

9.Cool in the freezer for approximately 10-20 minutes.

10.Remove liner and ENJOY!

28. <u>Coconut Whipped Cream with Berries</u>

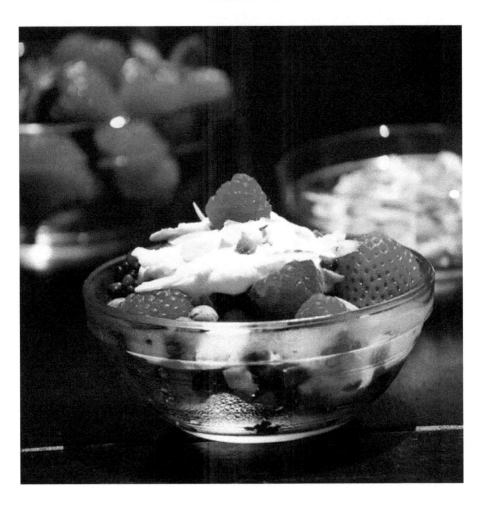

Ingredients:

- 2 cans of full fat coconut milk (cream only), chilled overnight
- 3-4 tablespoons pure maple syrup
- 3 teaspoons vanilla extract

- ½ teaspoon almond extract
- ½-1 teaspoon pumpkin pie spice
- Fresh organic berries to top

Directions:

1.To get started, you will want to chill your cans of coconut milk in the fridge for at least 6 hours, preferably overnight. When you remove the chilled can, be careful not to shake it.

2.Carefully open the can of coconut milk and scoop the thickened cream into a bowl, leaving behind the liquid coconut water.

3.Add the pure maple syrup, vanilla extract, almond extract, and pumpkin pie spice to the heavy coconut cream. Mix thoroughly with a hand mixer – will take 3-5 minutes for peaks to form.

4.Serve immediately or keep in the refrigerator to allow it to set more.

29. <u>Chocolate Hazelnut Cookies</u>

Ingredients:

- 1 cup whole raw hazelnuts or pecans
- ¼ cup coconut flour
- ½ teaspoon baking soda
- 2 dried Medjool dates (pitted)
- ½ teaspoon vanilla extract
- ⅓ cup whole raw almonds
- ¼ cup raw cacao powder
- ⅛ teaspoon sea salt
- ¼ cup softened virgin coconut oil
- 1-2 teaspoons raw honey

Directions:

1.Preheat oven to 350 degrees.

2.In a food processor, grind hazelnuts or pecans until coarse.

3.Add almonds and blend until nuts release just a bit of oil.

4.Add coconut flour and pulse.

5.Add cocoa powder and pulse.

6.Add baking soda and sea salt. Pulse again; the mixture should feel like fine

flour.

7.Transfer the dry ingredients to a bowl. Clean out food processor.

8.In empty food processor, add dates, coconut oil, raw honey and vanilla. Pulse until well incorporated.

9.Mix together the dry and wet mixtures.

10.Form small balls and gently press down into a cookie sheet lined with parchment paper.

11.Bake at 350 degrees for 8-10 minutes

30. <u>Cherry Walnut Balls</u>

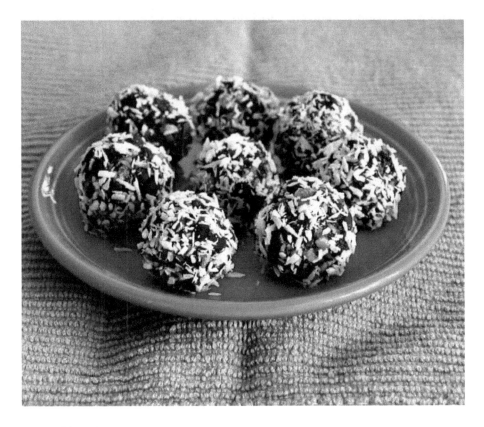

Ingredients:

- 1 cup (224 g) omega-3-rich margarine
- ¼ cup (6 g) sugar substitute
- ½ teaspoon vanilla extract
- 2¼ cups (270 g) all-purpose flour
- ¼ teaspoon salt
- ¼ teaspoon salt
- 1½ cups (88 g) walnuts, finely chopped

- ½ cup (60 g) dried cherries, finely chopped
- ½ cup (50 g) confectioners' sugar

Directions:

1. Preheat oven to 350°F (180°C, or gas mark 4).
2. In a large bowl, beat together the margarine, sugar substitute, and vanilla until creamy.
3. Slowly stir in the flour and salt until well blended. Stir in walnuts and dried cherries.
4. Shape into 1-inch (2.5-cm) balls and place on a cookie sheet lined with parchment paper.
5. Bake 13 to 15 minutes, until cookies are lightly browned on the bottom.
6. Remove from oven and set aside for 2 to 3 minutes, until cool enough to handle. Place the confectioners' sugar in a shallow dish. Roll the cookies in the confectioners' sugar while still warm, then set aside to cool.

31. <u>Apple Cherry Walnut Pie</u>

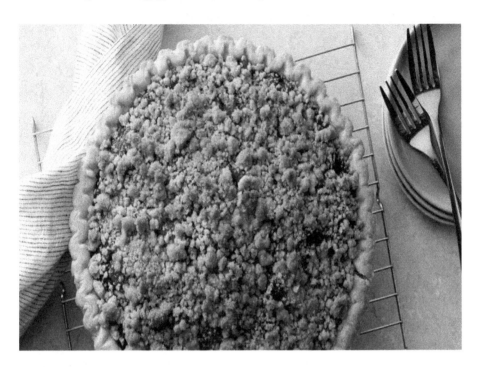

Ingredients:

For the crust:

- ½ cup (60 g) all-purpose flour
- ½ cup (60 g) whole-wheat flour
- ¼ cup (30 g) flaxseed, ground
- ¼ teaspoon salt
- ½ cup (112 g) omega-3-rich margarine
- 6 tablespoons (84 ml) cold water
- Canola oil spray

For the filling:

- 5 apples, cored and chopped
- 1 cup (125 g) dried cherries, chopped
- 1 cup (125 g) dried cherries, chopped
- ½ cup (12 g) sugar substitute

For the topping:

- ⅔ cup (80 g) whole-wheat flour
- ¼ cup (6 g) sugar substitute
- ¼ cup (55 g) brown sugar
- ½ cup (60 g) walnuts, chopped
- 1 teaspoon ground cinnamon
- ¼ teaspoon ground cloves
- 6 tablespoons (80 g) omega-3-rich margarine

1. Directions:
2. To make the crust: In a large bowl, mix together the flours, flaxseed, and salt.
3. Mix in the margarine, using a fork to blend, until the mixture resembles coarse crumbs.
4. Sprinkle a little water at a time on the dough, until it is moist enough to form into a ball. Flatten the dough ball on a lightly floured surface, and roll out to about 12 inches (30 cm) in diameter.
5. Preheat oven to 375°F (190°C, or gas mark 5). Lightly spray a 9-inch (22.5-cm) deep-dish pie pan with canola oil, and sprinkle with flour.

6. Lay the dough into the pie pan.

7. To make the filling: In a large bowl, stir together the apples, dried cherries, and sugar substitute. Spoon into the pie pan. Mix together the topping ingredients, and pour over the apple mixture.

8. Bake 50 to 55 minutes, until the top is golden brown.

32. <u>Cherry Blueberry Flambé</u>

Ingredients:

- ½ cup (12 g) sugar substitute
- 2 tablespoons (16 g) cornstarch
- ¼ cup (60 ml) cold water
- ¼ cup (60 ml) orange juice
- ½ teaspoon orange zest
- ½ teaspoon orange zest
- 1 pound (455 g) dark, sweet cherries, pitted
- 1 pint (300 g) blueberries
- 1 teaspoon vanilla extract
- ⅓ cup (80 ml) brandy or kirsch
- 3 cups (450 g) low-fat frozen yogurt
- ⅓ cup (50 g) whole almonds, toasted

Directions:

1. Mix sugar substitute with cornstarch in a medium-size saucepan. Add cold water and mix until dry ingredients are completely dissolved.
2. Blend in orange juice and orange zest.
3. Bring mixture to a boil over medium-high heat, whisking constantly until it is thickened.
4. Stir in the cherries, blueberries, and vanilla, reduce heat, and simmer 5 to 8 minutes, stirring gently.

5. Warm brandy in a separate saucepan. When ready to serve, transfer the cherry-blueberry sauce into a decorative casserole dish.
6. Pour the warm brandy or kirsch over the top and ignite.
7. When blue flame goes out, spoon over frozen yogurt in dessert dishes. Decorate with whole almonds, and serve.

33. __Chocolate Tofu Pudding__

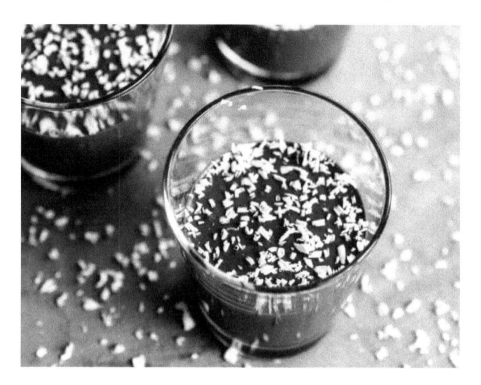

Ingredients:

- 6 ounces (170 g) bittersweet chocolate, chopped
- ¼ cup (30 g) unsweetened cocoa powder
- ½ cup (120 ml) water
- One 16-ounce (455 g) package firm tofu
- ¼ cup (60 ml) soy milk
- ¼ cup (60 ml) soy milk
- 1 tablespoon (14 ml) vanilla extract
- 8 ounces (225 g) fresh strawberries
- 1 banana

Directions:

1. Melt the chocolate, cocoa powder, and water over a double boiler. Set aside to cool.

2. In a blender or food processor, combine tofu, melted chocolate, soy milk, and vanilla extract. Process until the mixture is smooth and creamy.

3. Pour into individual pudding dishes, and place in the refrigerator to chill for 1½ to 2 hours.

4. Slice and quarter strawberries and banana. Serve over pudding.

34. __Dark Chocolate Strawberry Shortcake__

Ingredients:

- 2 cups (240 g) all-purpose flour
- ½ cup (125 g) unsweetened baking cocoa powder, divided
- 1 cup (25 g) sugar substitute, divided
- 2 teaspoons baking powder
- ½ teaspoon baking soda
- ¼ teaspoon salt
- ¼ cup (55 g) omega-3-rich margarine
- ⅓ cup (60 g) miniature chocolate chips ½ cup (120 ml) fat-free half-and-half
- ¼ cup (60 g) plain nonfat yogurt
- 4 pints (1.4 kg) strawberries, stemmed and sliced, divided
- Nonfat whipped topping

Directions:

1. Preheat oven to 400°F (200°C, or gas mark 6).
2. In a large bowl, mix together the flour, cocoa powder, ½ cup (12 g) sugar substitute, baking powder, soda, and salt.
3. Add the margarine and mash with a fork, until the mixture forms coarse crumbs.
4. Add the chocolate chips, half-andhalf,
5. and yogurt.

6. Mix until the dough forms a ball. Place the dough on a lightly floured surface, and knead until smooth. Roll out to about 1-inch (2.5-cm) thick.

7. Using a 2-inch (5-cm) round cookie cutter, cut out 12 to 15 shortcakes.

8. Line a cookie sheet with parchment paper. Place the shortcakes on the parchment paper and bake for 15 minutes. Remove from oven and set aside to cool.

9. Place 2 cups (220 g) of the strawberries and remaining sugar substitute in a blender or food processor. Process until smooth. Mix with the remaining strawberries in a medium-size bowl.

10. Cut the shortcakes in half, place a spoonful of nonfat whipped topping between the 2 halves, and serve topped with the strawberry topping.

35. __Chocolate Walnut Brownie__

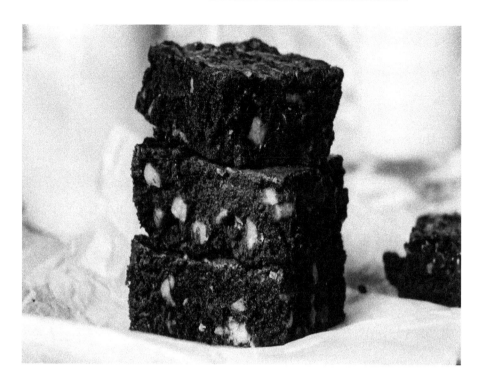

Ingredients:

For the brownies:

- Canola oil spray
- 4 squares (1 ounce [28 g] each) unsweetened chocolate
- ½ cup (100 g) puréed prunes
- 3 egg whites
- 2 tablespoons (28 ml) plus 1 teaspoon (5 ml) nonfat milk
- 2 tablespoons (28 ml) plus 1 teaspoon (5 ml) nonfat milk
- 2 tablespoons (28 ml) canola oil
- 1 teaspoon vanilla extract

- ¼ teaspoon salt
- 1½ cups (37 g) sugar substitute
- ¾ cup (90 g) all-purpose flour, sifted
- ½ cup (60 g) walnuts, chopped
- ½ cup (88 g) chocolate chips

For the sauce:

- 6 ounces (170 g) fresh or frozen raspberries, thawed
- ⅛cup (3 g) sugar substitute
- 1 tablespoon (14 ml) lemon juice
- 1 tablespoon (14 ml) water
- 1 tablespoon (14 ml) raspberry-flavored liqueur

For the topping:

- 1 cup (200 g) nonfat whipped topping, optional

Directions:

1. To make the brownies: Preheat oven to 350°F (180°C, or gas mark 4).
2. Spray the bottom of a 9 13-inch (22.5 × 32.5-cm) pan with canola oil. Melt the chocolate and puréed prunes in a double boiler, stirring occasionally.
3. Whisk together the egg whites, nonfat milk, and canola oil in a medium-size mixing bowl.
4. Add vanilla and salt. Stir in the sugar substitute and flour, and blend with the chocolate mixture.

5. Add the walnuts and chocolate chips. Spread evenly into baking pan.
6. Bake for 30 minutes. Allow brownies to cool before cutting into
7. squares.
8. To make the sauce: While brownies are cooking, prepare the sauce by combining all of the ingredients in a food processor or blender.
9. Process until smooth. Drizzle sauce over brownies and top with a dollop of nonfat whipped topping, if desired.

36. <u>Fruity Peppernuts</u>

Ingredients:

- 1 cup (225 g) brown sugar
- 1 cup (25 g) sugar substitute
- ¼ cup (55 g) omega-3-rich margarine
- 4 egg whites
- 1 cup (245 g) yogurt
- ¼ cup (75 g) unsweetened applesauce
- 1 teaspoon vanilla
- ½ pound (225 g) pitted dates, finely chopped
- 1 cup (125 g) walnuts, finely chopped
- 1 teaspoon baking powder
- 1 teaspoon baking soda
- 2 teaspoons cinnamon
- 1 teaspoon nutmeg
- 1 teaspoon allspice
- 3 cups (360 g) whole-wheat flour
- ½ cup (60 g) flaxseed, ground
- Canola oil spray

Directions:

1. Cream together brown sugar, sugar substitute, and margarine. Add egg whites and beat well.
2. Blend in yogurt, applesauce, and vanilla.

3. Stir in dates and walnuts until well mixed.

4. In a separate bowl, mix together remaining dry ingredients.

5. Using a spoon, add small amounts of the dry mixture to the batter, mixing well until a soft dough is formed.

6. Chill overnight in the refrigerator.

7. Preheat oven to 350°F (180°C, or gas mark 4). Divide dough into 3-inch (7.5- cm) balls. Roll each ball into a rope on a smooth, floured surface.

8. Using a dull knife, cut the rope into ½-inch (1-cm) pieces, about the size of a small nut.

9. Place on a baking sheet sprayed with canola oil and bake 10 to 12 minutes, or until golden brown.

37. <u>Dark Chocolate Almond Mousse</u>

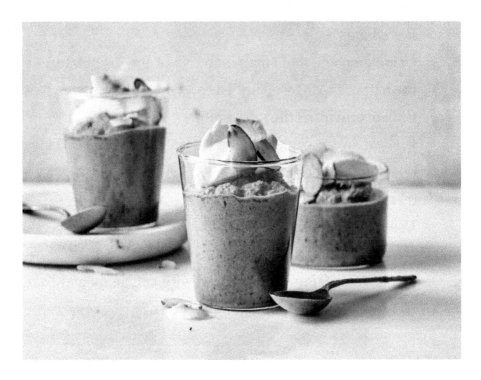

Ingredients:

- 6 ounces (170 g) 60-percent cacao bittersweet chocolate
- Pinch of salt
- 3 tablespoons (45 ml) hot water
- 1 tablespoon (15 ml) canola oil
- 1 tablespoon (15 ml) almond extract
- ¼ cup (30 g) unsweetened cocoa powder
- ¼ cup (6 g) sugar substitute
- ¼ cup (60 ml) nonfat milk
- 1 teaspoon unflavored gelatin

- 2 egg whites
- 1 cup (200 g) nonfat whipped topping
- ¼ cup (35 g) whole almonds, lightly toasted

Directions:

1. Melt the chocolate and salt in a double boiler, stirring often. Remove from heat.
2. Add in hot water, canola oil, and almond extract, and blend well. Blend in cocoa powder and sugar substitute.
3. Pour milk into a separate small bowl and sprinkle gelatin over until it absorbs the liquid.
4. Stir milk and gelatin until well blended,and add to the chocolate mixture.
5. Reheat the chocolate mixture over the double boiler, stirring constantly, until it is completely smooth. Remove from heat and allow to cool to room temperature.
6. In a small bowl, beat the egg whites until stiff peaks form. With a spatula, carefully fold in the egg whites into the cooled chocolate mixture, combining just until well blended.
7. Do not overmix.
8. Pour the mousse mixture into individual dessert dishes or ramekins, and refrigerate 1 to 2 hours until the mousse is set.
9. Decorate each serving with nonfat whipped topping and a few toasted almonds.

38. <u>Cranberry-Nut Truffles</u>

Ingredients:

- 2 cups (350 g) bittersweet chocolate, finely chopped
- One 8-ounce (225 g) package fat-free cream cheese
- 2½ cups (62 g) sugar substitute
- 1 cup (150 g) orange-flavored, sweetened dried cranberries, finely chopped 2
- cups (250 g) walnuts, finely chopped
- cups (250 g) walnuts, finely chopped
- ¼ cup (30 g) unsweetened cocoa powder

Directions:

1. Melt chocolate in a double boiler, and set aside to cool. In a large bowl, beat cream cheese until smooth.
2. Gradually beat in sugar substitute.
3. Stir in melted chocolate and dried cranberries, and blend well. Refrigerate 1 to 1½ hours.
4. Place chopped walnuts in a pie pan or shallow dish, and cocoa powder in a seconddish.
5. Remove chocolate mixture from refrigerator and shape into 1-inch (2.5-cm) balls, rolling each one in the chopped walnuts first, and then the cocoa powder, until evenly coated.

6. Store between layers of waxed paper in an airtight container in the refrigerator until ready to serve.

39. **Chocolate Cream Roll**

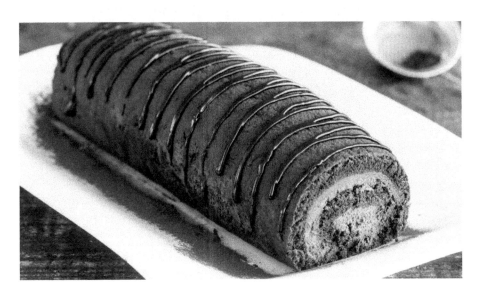

Ingredients:

For the filling:

- 1 egg white
- 1 cup (25 g) sugar substitute
- 3 tablespoons (40 ml) cold water
- 1 teaspoon cream of tartar
- 1 tablespoon (15 ml) melted dark chocolate
- 1 tablespoon (15 ml) melted dark chocolate
- ¼ cup (45 g) dark chocolate, finely chopped, optional

For the roll:

- 6 tablespoons (45 g) all-purpose flour
- 6 tablespoons (45 g) cocoa powder

- ½ teaspoon baking powder
- ¼ teaspoon salt
- 4 egg whites
- ¾ cup (18 g) plus 1 tablespoon (1.5 g) sugar substitute, divided 1 teaspoon vanilla extract
- 2½ tablespoons (35 ml) canola oil
- 3 tablespoons (40 ml) soy milk

Directions:

1. To make the filling: In a heat-resistant bowl, mix egg white, sugar substitute, cold water, and cream of tartar.
2. Place bowl over a pan of boiling water, and beat with a rotary beater until it stands in peaks.
3. Remove from heat and mix in melted dark chocolate and dark chocolate pieces. Set aside.
4. To make the roll: Preheat oven to 400°F (200°C, or gas mark 6).
5. Sift together flour, cocoa powder, baking powder, and salt in a large mixing bowl.
6. In a separate bowl, beat egg whites until stiff. Blend in ¾ cup (18 g) sugar substitute, vanilla, canola oil, and soy milk to egg whites. Stir into flour mixture.
7. Blend well.
8. Line a shallow 9 × 13-inch (22.5 × 32.5-cm) pan with parchment paper. Pour batter into pan.

9. Bake for 15 minutes. Remove from oven and carefully lift the parchment paper out of the pan.
10. Sprinkle lightly with 1 tablespoon (1.5 g) sugar substitute.
11. Cut off hard crusts. Spread filling evenly over chocolate roll, and roll up.
12. Place on a serving dish, seam side down. Serve sliced.

40. <u>Kiwi Pecan Pear Crisp</u>

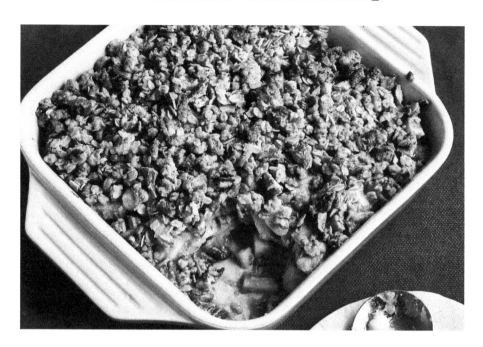

Ingredients:

For the crisp:

- 8 pears, cored and thinly sliced
- ¼ cup (40 g) raisins
- 2 kiwifruit, peeled and quartered
- 1 tablespoon (14 ml) lemon juice
- ½ teaspoon lemon zest
- ¼ cup (30 g) all-purpose flour
- ¼ cup (30 g) pecans, chopped
- ½ cup (12 g) sugar substitute

For the topping:

- ⅓ cup (75 g) omega-3-rich margarine
- ¼ cup (85 g) honey
- 1½ cups (112 g) rolled oats
- ½ cup (60 g) whole-wheat flour
- ½ teaspoon salt
- ½ teaspoon ground cinnamon
- ¼ teaspoon nutmeg
- ¼ teaspoon cloves

Directions:

1. To make the crisp: Preheat oven to 375°F (190°C, or gas mark 5).
2. In a large mixing bowl, combine the pears, raisins, kiwifruit, lemon juice, and lemon zest.
3. Toss gently, and add the flour.
4. Mix the pecans and sugar substitute in a separate bowl, and carefully combine with the pear mixture. Place in a shallow baking dish.
5. To make the topping: Melt the margarine and honey together.
6. Combine with the remaining topping ingredients and mix well.

7. Spread the topping evenly over the pear mixture. Place dish on the middle rack in the oven. Bake until top is golden brown, about 45 minutes.

41. <u>**Peach-Berry Port Wine Gelatin**</u>

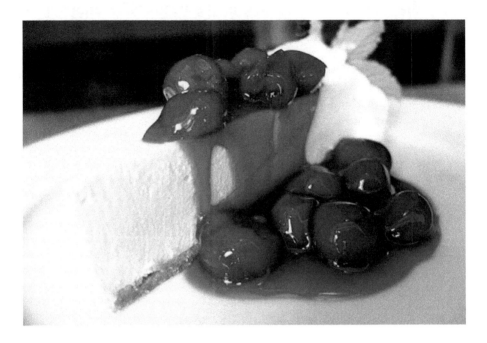

Ingredients:

- 1½ cups (355 ml) pomegranate juice, at room temperature
- 1 envelope plain gelatin
- ½ cup (120 ml) water
- ¾ cup (18 g) sugar substitute
- ½ cup (120 ml) port wine
- ½ cup (120 ml) port wine
- 1 pint (220 g) fresh raspberries, blackberries, or blueberries
- 1 cup (110 g) fresh strawberries, sliced
- 1 to 2 fresh peaches, sliced

Directions:

1. Nonfat whipped topping and fresh mint for garnish, optional
2. Pour pomegranate juice into a small mixing bowl, and sprinkle the gelatin over the top.
3. Do not stir the mixture because this can cause the gelatin to form lumps.
4. Set aside for 5 minutes. Meanwhile, mix together water and sugar substitute.
5. Set the bowl of gelatin over a pan of simmering water and heat, stirring occasionally, until the gelatin is completely dissolved. Add sugar substitute mixture and port wine. Continue to heat, stirring occasionally, until the liquid clarifies.
6. Pour a thin layer (about ½ inch [1 cm]) of the liquid into a medium-size to large gelatin mold. Chill until set, leaving remaining gelatin at room temperature.
7. Remove the mold from the refrigerator, and place raspberries and blueberries decoratively on top of the gelatin.
8. Pour enough gelatin over the berries to just cover them.
9. Chill again until set. Remove from the refrigerator and place the

10. peach and strawberry slices alternately on top of the set gelatin. Pour remaining gelatin over the fruit and chill until set.
11. Remove mold from refrigerator, and place in a container of hot water just below the edge of the mold.
12. Allow mold to sit for 30 seconds before inverting
13. over a serving plate.
14. Serve as is, or with nonfat whipped topping and mint leaves.

42. <u>Pecan Cakes with Raspberry Sauce</u>

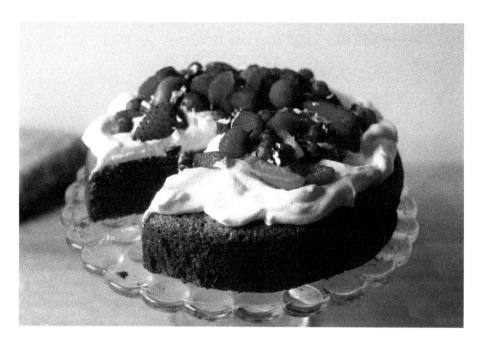

For the cakes:

- Canola oil cooking spray
- ¾ cup (75 g) pecans, toasted
- ½ cup (112 g) omega-3-rich margarine
- ½ cup (125 g) unsweetened applesauce
- 1 cup (25 g) sugar substitute
- ½ cup (100 g) granulated sugar
- ½ cup (100 g) granulated sugar
- 1 teaspoon vanilla
- 4 egg whites
- 2½ teaspoons baking powder

- ½ teaspoon salt
- ½ cup (60 g) whole-wheat flour
- 1½ cups (180 g) all-purpose flour
- ¼ cup (30 g) ground flaxseed
- 1¼ cups (295 ml) soy milk

For the sauce:

- ¼ cup (60 ml) apple juice
- 1 cup (25 g) sugar substitute
- 1 tablespoon (8 g) cornstarch
- 2 cups (220 g) fresh raspberries
- 1 teaspoon orange zest

Directions:

1. Preheat oven to 350°F (180°C, or gas mark 4). Lightly spray and flour 2 muffin or tart pans.
2. Process pecans in a food processor to a medium-fine grind. Set
3. aside.
4. To make the cakes: In a large mixing bowl, blend margarine, applesauce, sugar substitute, and sugar. Add vanilla and egg whites.
5. In a separate bowl, combine the dry ingredients. Add the pecans and mix well.
6. Add flour mixture and soy milk alternately to the margarine mixture, blending after each addition.

7. Beat the batter on low speed until well blended. Spoon the batter into tart or muffin pans.
8. Bake 15 to 20 minutes, or until a wooden toothpick inserted into the cakes comes out clean.
9. Cool for 5 minutes, and remove from pans.
10. To make the sauce: Heat the apple juice and sugar substitute in a small saucepan.
11. Once the sauce boils, add the cornstarch, stir well, and turn the heat to low.
12. Simmer 5 to 10 minutes, until the sauce thickens. Remove from heat.
13. Stir in fresh raspberries and orange zest, reserving a few raspberries for the garnish.
14. Top cakes with raspberry sauce and garnish with fresh raspberries.

Lightning Source UK Ltd.
Milton Keynes UK
UKHW020717270521
384465UK00005B/238